Complete Keto Dinner Cookbook

Tasty and Healthy Recipes for Women Over 50, to End the day in the Right way

Katie Attanasio

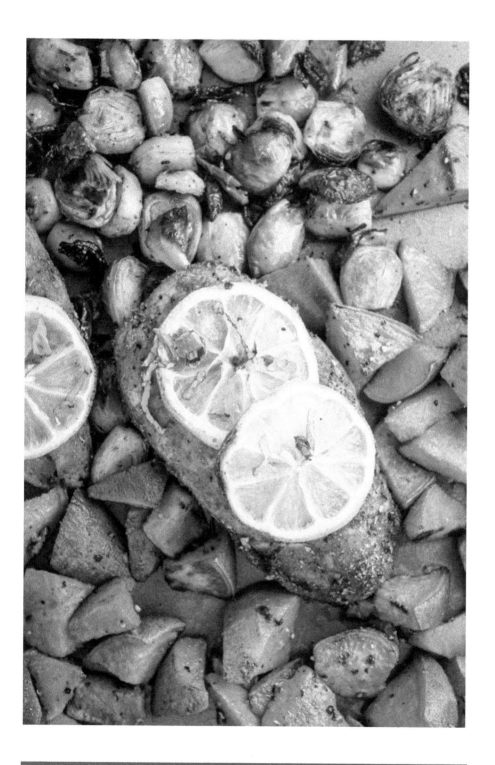

© Copyright 2021 - All rights reserved.

Table of Contents

50 Tasty Dinner Recipes

1   Keto Instant Pot Cabbage Rolls

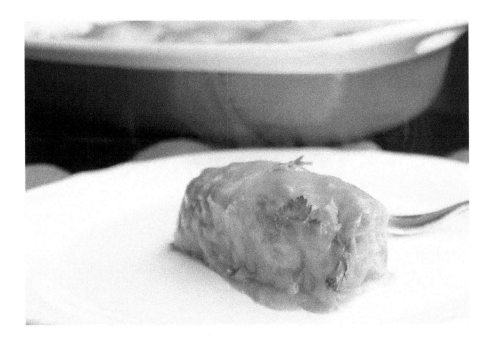

Servings: 12 | **Time:** 1 hr 20 mins | **Difficulty**: Easy

Nutrients per serving: Calories: 218 kcal | Fat: 14g | Carbohydrates: 6g | Protein: 14g | Fiber: 2g

Ingredients

1 cup of water

One head cabbage

FILLING:

1 pound ground Pork

1 pound ground beef

2 tsp onion powder

1 tsp garlic powder

2 tsp finely chopped parsley

2 tsp salt

½ tsp pepper

1 tbsp Worcestershire

One big egg

SAUCE:

2 tbsp additional-virgin olive oil

2 tsp dried oregano

1/2 chopped cup onion Three minced cloves garlic

2 tbsp tomato paste

28 ounces canned crushed tomatoes

1 tbsp Worcestershire

1 tsp Salt

Method

1.   On med boil, heat the olive oil in a frying pan.

2.   Put the onions when the olive oil is hot and cook for 2 mins. Put the garlic & cook for another min to finish cooking.

3.   Put the leftover sauce ingredients mix together for around 15-20 mins, cooking on med heat, stirring periodically, while the stuffed cabbage is being cooked.

FILLING:

1.   In a big bowl, mix all the filling ingredients & work them together with the hands.

2.   Until going on to the next move, wash your hands carefully.

3.   Assemble rolls of cabbage.

4.   With the lid on, fill a pot big enough to accommodate your cabbage. Get things to a boil with a kettle of water.

5.   Core your cabbage & put it in the water. Cover it with a lid.

6.   For 5-7 mins, cook.

7.   Take the cabbage from water & peel off the cabbage's head with a pliable cabbage leaf & position it on the flat surface.

8.	At the end of a leaf, put 3 ounces of the meat combination along with the stem.

9.	If you roll the leaf on the meat, fold it into the side of the cabbage leaf & begin rolling till the end is reached.

COOK IN THE INSTANT POT/COOKER Under PRESSURE:

1.	In the Slow Cooker Insert, put a trivet & place one cup of water into the rim.

2.	Put on the trivet for the first cabbage rolls and cover with 1 cup of sauce.

3.	Put the 2nd row of cabbage rolls in different directions on top of the 1st row. Put 1 cup of sauce.

4.	Repeat & top with the leftover sauce for a third coat, allowing it to spill down the sides of cabbage rolls to cover everything.

5.	Secure the cover in place & set up the SEALING valve. Set to HIGH PRESSURE for 20 mins & cook.

6.	Before carefully moving the valve to vent & allowing the residual steam to escape, allow the Instant Pot to perform a natural release for fifteen min after it has done.

7.	From the jar, extract the stuffed cabbage & put it aside.

8.	Set the Instant Pot to sauté & boil the sauce in the pot, stirring continuously—Cook for ten min or till thickened to a pasta sauce's consistency.

9.	Plate a stuffed cabbage in a wide bowl. Now enjoy it.

2   Instant Pot Chicken Bone Broth

Servings: 12 | **Time:** 2 hrs 30 mins | **Difficulty**: Easy

Nutrients per serving: Calories: 45 kcal | Fat: 1g | Carbohydrates: 1g | Protein: 5g

Ingredients

4 Chicken Wings

2 Rotisserie Chicken carcasses

2 roughly chopped stalks Celery

1 roughly chopped Carrot

1 big quartered Onion

1 bunch fresh thyme

2 Bay Leaves

2 to 3 sprigs Fresh Rosemary

2 tsp Salt

½ tsp Pepper Water

Method

1.   In the Slow Cooker, put all the ingredients & fill the pot with water till it reaches just below the peak fill mark.

2.   Turn the valve on top to SEALING & set the Slow Cooker to HIGH pressure for 120 mins. Lock the Instant Pot lid in position.

3.   Click CANCEL when the timer goes off & then allow it to make a natural release for thirty min.

4.   After thirty min, flip your valve to VENTING to clear the lid & let out some residual steam.

5.   To strain the vegetables, herbs & chicken bones, spill the broth into a bowl via a fine mesh strainer. Add salt

6.   Please place it in a sealed jar in the fridge. Till ready for usage, or ice for up to six months in a sealed jar.

3   Keto Chicken Parmesan Roll-Ups

Servings: 10 | **Time:** 1 hr 10 mins | **Difficulty:** Easy

Nutrients per serving: Calories: 155 kcal | Fat: 9g | Carbohydrates: 5g | Protein: 15g | Fiber: 2g

Ingredients

Two full aubergine

16 ounces chicken breast, Cooked & shredded

1 tbsp Italian seasoning

1 tsp Salt

2 cups divided Rao's Marinara Sauce

½ cup Mozzarella Cheese

1 cup Parmesan cheese

Method

1.   Oven preheated to 210 degrees C.

2.   Carefully slice the aubergine into long vertical slices that are ¼ inch wide by using a mandolin.

3.   Layer the slices in a single layer on a cookie sheet lined with bakery release paper. Cook 12 to 15 mins. This move is to dry the aubergine such that it does not leak a lot of water when it heats, so it is finished as it seems that any have shrunk & are partially dry and not brown/burned.

4.   Take it from the oven when the aubergine has completed baking & let it cool for 10 mins.

5.   Lower the temperature of the oven.

6.   Mix the chopped chicken, Italian Seasoning, 1⁄4 cup of marinara sauce, Parmesan cheese, & salt in a wide bowl while the aubergine is cooling.

7.   To the bottom of even an oven-safe baking dish, apply half a cup of marinara.

8.   At one end of an aubergine strip, put roughly 2.5 ounces of chopped chicken combination & roll it up gently. Put the roll with the overlapping end face down in the baking dish. For any of the aubergine slices, repeat this.

9.   Top with two teaspoons of marinara sauce for each aubergine roll. Drizzle the mozzarella cheese on the rolls & put for 20 mins in the oven to roast.

4 Provolone And Prosciutto Stuffed Pork Loin

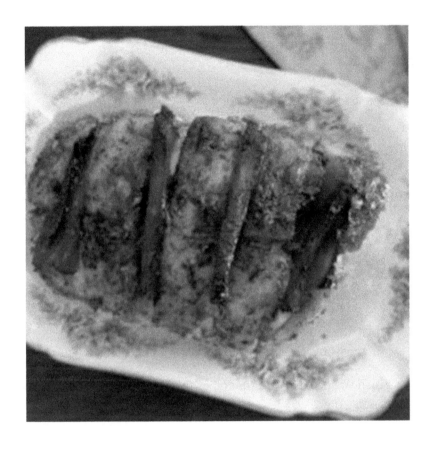

Servings: 10 | **Time**: 1 hr 15 mins | **Difficulty**: Easy

Nutrients per serving: Calories: 323 kcal | Fat: 18g | Carbohydrates: 1g | Protein: 37g | Fiber: 1g

Ingredients

3 pounds trimmed Pork loin

6 ounces Prosciutto

6 slices Provolone

1 tbsp Olive Oil

3 tsp Salt

2 tsp Pepper

Method

1.   oven preheated to 400 degrees.

2.   Trim the pork loin's excess fat & butterfly it.

3.   On the open pork loin, put the provolone slices & then finish with sliced prosciutto.

4.   "Safe roast tightly spaced 1 to 2 apart with butcher's twine.

5.   Brush with olive oil on the top of the pork loin & drizzle with salt & ground pepper.

6.   Bake & cover for 45 mins. Then cut the foil & resume cooking for ten min or till the internal temp has reached 80 degrees C.

7.   Take it from the oven before cutting the twine & slicing, then allow the roast to stand for ten mins.

5   Low Carb Pizza Casserole

Servings: 10 | **Time:**1 hr 15 mins | **Difficulty:** Easy

Nutrients per serving: Calories: 519 kcal | Fat: 43g | Carbohydrates: 7g | Protein: 27g | Fiber: 3g

Ingredients

ounces Pepperoni

14 ounces Cauliflower florets

2 pounds Italian Sausage

1 tbsp Olive Oil

8 ounces sliced Mushrooms

1 Green Pepper

12 ounces shredded Mozzarella cheese

1.5 cups Low Carb Pasta Sauce

1/4 cup powdered Parmesan cheese

1 tsp Italian Seasoning

Method

1.   steam your cauliflower. In a safe microwave bowl with one cup of water, put the cut cauliflower. Cover with a wet paper towel & microwave for around 3 mins or till the cauliflower is soft.

2.   Drain your cauliflower with a towel.

3.   Oven preheated to 200 degrees C

4.   Cook the Italian sausage in a big pan over med heat for around 15 mins. Drain the extra fat once the sausage has done cooking.

5.   Put the olive oil & sauté the mushrooms for ten min on med-high heat to extract the excess water in the same saucepan.

6.   Coat it with non-stick spray. Prepare a 13 to a 9-inch baking dish and then spread 1/2 cup of pasta sauce on the bottom.

7.   Place the cooked Italian sausage, cauliflower, green peppers & mushrooms in a wide dish. Toss together once blended well.

8.   In the baking dish, spread ½ of the combination. Cover with ½ cup of pasta sauce, accompanied by ½ cup of pepperoni & then 6 ounces of mozzarella cheese.

9.   Then spread the leftover combination of toppings over the egg, accompanied by the pepperonis, the remaining ½ cup of pasta sauce, & Six ounces mozzarella cheese.

10.   Mix the Italian Seasoning & parmesan cheese in a tiny bowl.

11.   Drizzle over the casserole with the Parmesan combination & finish with Ten pepperoni slices.

12.   Put the cheese in the oven & cook for thirty min or till the casserole is fully cooked & the cheese is melted.

6   Keto Big Mac Casserole

Servings: 10 | **Time**: 50 mins | **Difficulty**: Easy

Nutrients per serving: Calories: 487 kcal | Fat: 41g | Carbohydrates: 5g | Protein: 25g | Fiber: 1g

Ingredients

½ cup diced Onion

2 pounds Ground beef

1 tbsp Worcestershire

2 tsp Garlic powder

2 tsp divided Salt

1 tsp divided Pepper

2 tbsp Dill pickle relish

2 ounces Cream cheese

Four big Eggs

8 ounces shredded Cheddar cheese

1/4 cup Heavy cream

BIG MAC SAUCE:

4 tbsp Dill pickle relish

1/2 cup Mayonnaise

2 tbsp Yellow mustard

1 tsp Paprika

1 tsp White wine vinegar

1 tsp Garlic powder

1 tsp Onion powder

Method

1.   Oven preheated to 175 degrees C.

2.   In a pan on med-high pressure, prepare the ground beef. Put the Worcestershire sauce, diced onions, garlic powder, 1 tsp & 1⁄2 tsp of pepper after cooking for around 7 mins. Continue cooking the ground beef for 3 mins or till the ground beef is completely cooked.

3.   Until putting the beef back in the skillet, move the ground beef to the strainer & let the excess fat drain out.

4.   To the ground beef, put the cream cheese & heat over med-low heat till your cream cheese is melted & the beef is covered.

5.   Mix in the dill relish & extract the combination from the heat.

6.   Scoop the beef combination into an 11-7 inch baking dish.

7.   Beat the heavy cream, eggs, 1 tsp of salt & 1⁄2 tsp of pepper together in a shallow bowl.

8.   Shake the baking dish softly and place the egg combination over the ground beef such that the egg combination is equally distributed.

9.   Cover with the grated cheese.

10.   For thirty min or till the casserole is set, put the dish in an oven to bake.

11.   The casserole dish gives the Large Mac sauce by stirring all the ingredients in the tiny bowl.

12.   Sprinkle it with a Big Mac sauce before serving as the casserole falls out of the oven.

7   Big Mac Keto Meatloaf

Servings: 8 | **Time:** 1 hr 25 mins | **Difficulty**: Easy

Nutrients per serving: Calories: 499 kcal | Fat: 40g | Carbohydrates: 4g | Protein: 30g | Fiber: 1g

Ingredients

KETO MEATLOAF:

2 pounds Ground beef

2 cup finely crushed Pork rinds

1 Egg

2 tsp Onion powder

2 tbsp Worcestershire sauce

1 tsp Salt

8 ounces American Cheese

½ tsp Garlic powder

BIG MAC SAUCE:

2 tbsp Dill pickle relish

1/4 cup Mayonnaise

1 tbsp Yellow mustard

1/2 tsp Paprika

½ tsp White wine vinegar

1/2 tsp Garlic powder

1/2 tsp Onion powder

Method

1.   Oven preheated to 175 degrees C.

2.   Mix the pork rinds, ground beef, egg, onion powder, Worcestershire sauce, salt & garlic powder in a big bowl. Mix the components till they're fully mixed.

3.   Press 1/2 of the ground beef combination onto the bottom of a loaf pan lined with bakery release paper. Leave a 1-inch lip to create a small indentation in the middle of the ground beef.

4.   Put the cubed American cheese in the indentation & press it into the bottom half with the leftover ground beef combination, so the meatloaf is covered.

5.   For 60 to 70 mins, bake.

6.   All the Big Mac sauce components are whisked together in a bowl as the meatloaf bakes.

7.   Take the meatloaf from the oven when you stop baking and let it rest for ten min.

8.   Take it from the pan & then line it with Big Mac sauce.

8   Italian Sausage And Pepper Foil Packet Meal

Servings: 6 | **Time:** 30 mins | **Difficulty:** Easy

Nutrients per serving: Calories: 553 kcal | Fat: 48g | Carbohydrates: 8g | Protein: 23g | Fiber: 2g

Ingredients

Two large dice Red Bell Peppers

2 pounds Italian Sausage

Two large dice Yellow Bell Peppers

One thinly sliced Red Onion

Pepper Salt

Method

1.   Cut the Italian sausage into strips.

2.   Cut the veggies into wedges.

3.   Mix the meat & veggies & put salt & pepper.

4.   Cover & barbecue in a foil packet for 20 mins or till the sausage has cooked through.

9   Chimichurri Steak

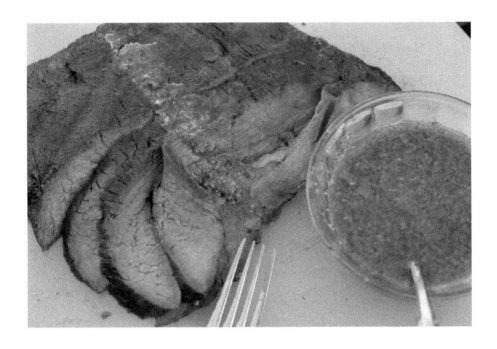

Servings: 6 | **Time**: 25 mins | **Difficulty:** Easy

Nutrients per serving: Calories: 395 kcal | Fat: 27g | Carbohydrates: 1g | Protein: 32g

Ingredients

2 pound Flank Steak

1/2 tsp Salt Chimichurri Sauce

1/2 tsp Pepper

Method

1.   Salt & pepper the flank steak gently & let it hang out & hit room temp.

2.   Heat the grill at 225 C.

3.   Make the chimichurri sauce, whereas the steak hits room temp & the barbecue heats up.

4.   Put the flank steak on the barbecue when the barbecue is prepared, & cook on each side for around five min or till the steak reaches an internal temp of 125 F - 145 F.

5.   Carry it in & let it rest for fifteen min till the steak is finished. Then break the beef into thin pieces & split through the grain.

6.   Put chimichurri sauce on top & enjoy!

10   Instant Pot Big Mac Soup

Servings: 8 | **Time:** 45 mins | **Difficulty:** Easy

Nutrients per serving: Calories: 492 kcal | Fat: 43g | Carbohydrates: 6g | Protein: 20g | Fiber: 1g

Ingredients

1 tbsp Butter

1 pound Ground Beef

1/2 cup diced Onion

1 cup diced Celery

1 finely minced clove Garlic

6 ounces thinly sliced Cabbage

1 big Dill pickle

1 tbsp Worcestershire sauce

1 cup Heavy cream

3 cups Beef broth

12 ounces American Cheese

Sesame Seeds for garnish

SPECIAL SAUCE:

4 tbsp Dill pickle relish

1/2 cup Mayonnaise

2 tbsp Yellow mustard

1 tsp Paprika

1 tsp White wine vinegar

1 tsp Garlic powder

1 tsp Onion powder

Method

1. Your ground beef is brown. Put ground beef & mix till browned. Set Instant Pot to SAUTE. Press cancel to end the saute feature

2. Drain the ground beef grease & return to the Instant Pot.

3. Put the celery, onion, cabbage, garlic, Worcestershire sauce, beef broth & dill pickle. Fasten the cover, place the pressure valve on top for SEALING & cook at HIGH PRESSURE for ten min.

4. Click cancel to finish the cooking when the timer goes off and leave for five min to release it naturally. Turning the valve to VENTING to relieve the remaining pressure.

5. Remove the cover of the Instant Pot & switch on the SAUTE feature. Put Heavy cream & American cheese, stirring till the cheese is fully melted.

6. Mix the special sauce ingredients in the tiny bowl.

7. Serve the soup with a topping of sesame seeds & a drizzle of a special sauce till the cheese has melted.

11 Low Carb Moo Shu Pork

Servings: 4 | **Time:** 2 hrs 11 mins | **Difficulty**: Easy

Nutrients per serving: Calories: 660 kcal | Fat: 60g | Carbohydrates: 7g | Protein: 13g | Fiber: 7g

Ingredients

1 pound pork, cut into thin pieces

4 Carb Balance tender

Taco Flour Tortillas

2 eggs

2 tbsp vegetable oil

5 ounces shiitake mushrooms

8 ounces slaw Mix

2 ounces bean sprouts

3 ounces bok choy

2 tbsp sliced scallions

MARINADE:

1 tsp fresh ginger

2 crushed cloves garlic

6 tbsp soy sauce

2 tbsp rice vinegar

1 tsp sesame oil

1 tsp five Spice Powder

HOISIN SAUCE:

1/2 teaspoon fresh ginger

3 to 5 drops liquid sweetener

2 tbsp black bean paste

3 tbsp soy sauce

1/2 tsp sesame oil

1 tbsp rice vinegar

1 tsp Sriracha hot sauce

1/2 tsp 5 spice powder

Method

1.   In a little bowl, mix all of the marinade ingredients. Divided in two.

2.   In the bowl, put the thinly sliced pork and add ½ of the marinade on the pork. Stir such that the meat is completely coated, then cover & allow to marinate for at least 2hrs in the freezer. Place the excess marinade in the refrigerator in a little jar till ready for usage.

3.   Mix the hoisin ingredients in a tiny bowl & put aside.

4.   In a shallow bowl, put the eggs together.

5.   On med-high heat, heat a wide skillet. Put 1 tbsp of marinated pork & vegetable oil. Cook for about five min, till most of the pork, is ready.

6.   Put the eggs into the skillet & proceed to mix, then cook for around 1 min, till the eggs are scrambled.

7.   Put the slaw mix, vegetable oil, bean sprouts, mushrooms, bok choy, & the reserved marinade to the second tbsp. Continue cooking for five min or till the

8.   Serve it with the extra bean sprouts, scallions to garnish, a sprinkle of low carb hoisin sauce & Moo Shu Pork. Heat the Project Carb Balance Tortillas for the greatest taste.

12   Instant Pot Butter Chicken

Servings: 8 | **Time:** 32 mins | **Difficulty:** Easy

Nutrients per serving: Calories: 394 kcal | Fat: 30g | Carbohydrates: 9g | Protein: 20g | Fiber: 2g

Ingredients

2 cups diced Onion

Five cloves minced Garlic

4 tbsp Butter

15 ounces Tomato sauce

2 pounds chicken thighs

2 tbsp Red curry paste

3 tbsp Tomato paste

1 1/2 tsp ground ginger 2

 tsp Garam masala

1 tsp Salt

½ tsp Smoked paprika

1/2 cup Heavy cream

Coriander for garnish

Method

1.   Put onion, garlic & butter, and prepare your Slow Cooker to SAUTE. Saute till the onions are soft, for about five min. Cancel the saute by pressing OFF.

2.   To the slow cooker, put the tomato sauce, chicken, tomato paste, garam masala, red curry paste, ground ginger, salt & smoked paprika. Close it with the lid in position & switch the pressure valve for 7 mins   at HIGH PRESSURE.

3.   Do the natural release for five min once the timer goes off & then move the valve over the top to VENTING to get the excess steam out from the pressure cooker.

4.   Take the cover off & extract the chicken from the sauce with a slotted spoon, and put it aside.

5.   Put the heavy cream in a pot &, till creamy, puree the sauce using the immersion blender.

6.   Set the slow cooker to SAUTE & mix the sauce for 7 to 10 mins till boiling, or till it thickens. Turn the Saute OFF.

7.   Return the chicken to the sauce, mix & serve with the coriander garnish.

13 Roasted Cauliflower Steaks With Brown Butter

Servings: 2 | **Time:** 5 mins | **Difficulty**: Easy

Nutrients per serving: Calories: 249 kcal | Fat: 23g | Carbohydrates: 9g | Protein: 4g | Fiber: 3g

Ingredients

¼ cup Olive Oil

2 heads Cauliflower

½ tsp Salt

½ cup salted Butter

4 tbsp capers

1 Lemon

½ Walnuts cup

Method

1.   oven preheated to10 degrees C.

2.   Cut cauliflower into "steaks" 1 inch deep.

3.   Brush the cauliflower steaks with oil of olive on both sides & put them on a cookie sheet. Do not use bakery release paper, or the lovely caramelization would not be obtained.

4.   Season with salt & bake for around 10 mins in the oven. Before flipping, the cauliflower must have a good brown color to it. Then flip for the next ten min and begin to roast.

5.   Make the brown butter as the cauliflower bakes. Put the butter on medium heat to a hot skillet.

6.   It will foam when the butter cooks, & then you would see tiny brown bits start developing on the bottom. It is finished till the color of the batter hits a rich golden-brown color. In the bowl, put in the brown butter. To remove brown bits from the bottom, you should strain the butter or not. It depends on you!

7.   On med heat, put the capers & walnuts in the pan & gently toast them for 2 to 3 mins. Then place   the brown butter again in the skillet.

8.   Take it from the oven & spoon the capers, walnuts & brown butter on the cauliflower steaks once the cauliflower has done baking.

9.   Squeeze lemon on your cauliflower & enjoy.

14 Sheet Pan Curried Chicken And Vegetables

Servings: 6 | **Time:** 40 mins | **Difficulty:** Easy

Nutrients per serving: Calories: 397 kcal | Fat: 28g | Carbohydrates: 14g | Protein: 21g | Fiber: 5g

Ingredients

4 tbsp divided Olive oil

4 tsp divided Curry powder

2 tsp divided Salt

3 cups Carrots

4 cups Cauliflower florets

2 Red bell peppers

1 tbsp shredded fresh ginger

6 Chicken thighs

2 cups chopped Green onions

1 cup finely chopped coriander

Method

1.   Oven preheated to 220 degrees C.

2.   Combine 2 tsp of curry powder, two tablespoons of olive oil, & 1 tsp of salt in a wide bowl. Put the carrots, cauliflower, bell pepper, and ginger, then toss gently till fully surrounded in a bowl.

3.   Arrange a greased/ lined sheet pan with the veggies.

4.   Put the leftover two tbsp of olive oil, 2 tsp of curry powder & 1 tsp in another cup. To the dish, put the chicken thighs & toss till it's covered.

5.   Put chicken thighs on the sheet pan above the veggies.

6.   Cook your chicken in an oven for 20 mins, extract it from the oven & sprinkle the chicken & veggies with the green onions. Put it back in the oven & proceed to bake for another ten mins or till the chicken is completely cooked.

7.   Sprinkle with coriander & take the tray from the oven.

15 Grilled Chicken Fajita Skewers

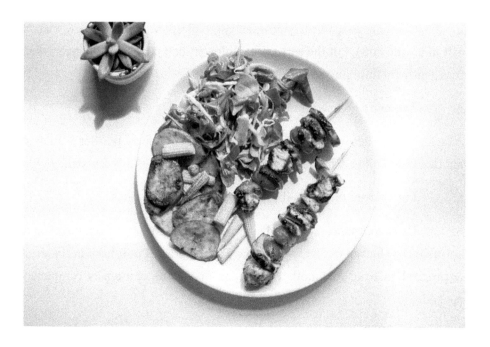

Servings: 4 | **Time:** 28 mins | **Difficulty**: Easy

Nutrients per serving: Calories: 195 kcal | Fat: 4g | Carbohydrates: 12g | Protein: 26g | Fiber: 4g

Ingredients

1 lb cubed Chicken Breast

3 Tbsp Chili powder

1/2 Tbsp Garlic powder

2 Tbsp Cumin

1/2 tsp salt plus extra to taste

1 Green Bell Pepper

1 Red Bell Pepper

1 Yellow Bell Pepper

1 Red Onion

Method

1.   Mix the garlic powder, chili powder, salt & cumin in a wide bowl.

2.   In spice mix, Put cubed chicken & toss till it's covered.

3.   On a skewer, alternate b/w peppers, onions & chicken till every skewer is filled.

4.   Sprinkle the skewers with a little extra salt.

5.   Grill 4 to 5 mins per side or till chicken is baked through, on med-high heat.

6.   Serve the fajitas with tortillas of corn/flour, salsa, sour cream, guacamole, & something else you want!

16 Fire Roasted Red Pepper Soup

Servings: 2 | **Time:** 5 mins | **Difficulty:** Easy

Nutrients per serving: Calories: 39 kcal | Carbohydrates: 8g | Protein: 1g | Fiber: 2g

Ingredients

28 oz canned Tomatoes

9 oz diced Onion

3 cloves Garlic

16 oz Roasted Red Peppers

2 Tbsp Tomato Paste

1/2 tsp Salt

2 c Broth, chicken/ vegetable

Method

1.   Saute the onions in a big pot on med heat till the onions are soft. Put the garlic & finish cooking for two min.

2.   Put the tomatoes, roasted red peppers, broth & tomato paste.

3.   Carry to a boil & then simmer it on low pressure & cover it.

4.   Cook for thirty mins.

5.   Just use the immersion blender to puree the soup components till the soup becomes smooth.

6.   .Sprinkle with salt to taste

17   Herb Crusted Grilled Leg Of Lamb

Servings: 10 | **Time:** 50 mins | **Difficulty**: Easy

Nutrients per serving: Calories: 273 kcal | Fat: 21g | Carbohydrates: 1g | Protein: 70g

Ingredients

2.5 lb butterflied & trimmed Aussie Boneless leg of lamb

4 minced Garlic cloves.

2 Tbsp juice of Lemon

1 Tbsp True Aussie Lamb Rub

½ c Parsley

6 Tbsp Unsalted softened butter

¼ c Coriander

Method

1.   heat barbecue to 175 degrees C.

2.   In the bowl, mix the rub, butter, garlic, parsley, coriander & lemon juice.

3.   Cover the lamb's butterfly leg in herbal butter.

4.   Put a leg of lamb on a barbecue & sear on each side for five min.

5.   Cover the barbecue lid & cook for 30 to 40 mins until the lamb's inside temp exceeds 130 degrees F.

6.   Take it off the barbecue & let it sit for ten mins. Slice & eat.

18   Keto Chicken Tenders

Servings: 2 | **Time**: 16 mins | **Difficulty**: Easy

Nutrients per serving: Calories: 474 kcal | Fat: 60g | Carbohydrates: 7g | Protein: 13g | Fiber: 7g

Ingredients

1 cup almond flour

8 ounces chicken breast tenderloins

1 tsp salt

1 tsp pepper

1 big egg

1/4 cup Heavy Whipping

Method

1.   Beat the egg & put milk in the big bowl to cover them. Sprinkle With salt & pepper. Put the chicken & let it rest for ten min.

2.   In a shallow dish/pan, put the almond flour & sprinkle with pepper & salt.

3.   Coat the chicken with flour on all ends.

4.   Fry till golden brown & the internal temperature exceeds 1600 in tiny batches. Dip in the favorite keto-friendly sauce of your choosing.

19 Keto Salisbury Steak With Mushroom Gravy

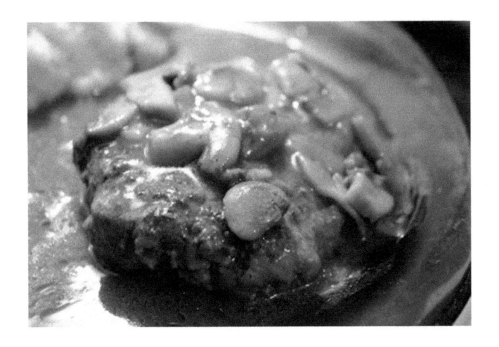

Servings: 6 | **Time:** 30 mins | **Difficulty:** Easy

Nutrients per serving: Calories: 457 kcal | Fat: 34g | Carbohydrates: 5g | Protein: 32g

Ingredients

For the Salisbury Steaks:

3/4 cup almond flour

2 lbs ground chuck

1 Tbsp chopped fresh parsley

1 Tbsp Worcestershire sauce

1/4 cup beef broth

1 Tbsp dried onion flakes

1/2 tsp garlic powder

1/2 tsp ground black pepper

1 1/2 tsp kosher salt

For the gravy:

2 Tbsp bacon grease

2 Tbsp butter

1 cup sliced yellow onions

2 cups sliced button mushrooms

1/2 cup beef broth

1/2 tsp Worcestershire sauce

salt & pepper

1/4 cup sour cream

Method

1.   In a med sized bowl, mix all the steak components & blend well.

2.   Shape into six oval patties around 1 inch thick & put on a baking sheet.

3.   Bake for 18 mins in the preheated 185 degrees (C) oven.

4.   In a wide skillet, melt the butter & bacon fat.

5.   Put the mushrooms & cook till golden brown on med heat (about 3 minutes per side.)

6.   Put the onions & simmer on med heat for five min, till golden & smooth.

7.   Put the Worcestershire sauce & broth, mix & simmer for 3 mins, stirring to brush off any pieces from the bottom of a pan.

8.   Stir well, put the sour cream & take it from the heat.

9.   Sprinkle with salt.

10.   If needed, serve on the hot Salisbury Steaks with additional parsley for topping.

20   One Pot Cheesy Taco Skillet

Servings: 6 | **Time:** 20 mins | **Difficulty:** Easy

Nutrients per serving: Calories: 341 kcal | Fat: 20g | Carbohydrates: 9g | Protein: 30g | Fiber: 1g

Ingredients

One large diced yellow onion

1 lb lean ground beef

2 diced bell peppers

1 large shredded courgette

1 can diced tomatoes with green chilis

3 cups baby kale or spinach combination taco

seasoning green

onions for garnish

1 1/2 cup shredded cheddar & jack cheese

Method

1.   In a wide skillet, put lightly brown beef & crumble it good.

2.   Drain the excess fat.

3.   Put the peppers & onions, then fry till browned.

4.   Put canned tomatoes, taco seasoning, as well, as any water required for taco seasoning to cover the combination evenly (up to 1 tbsp- the liquid from the tomatoes will help)

5.   Put the greens & leave to wilt absolutely.

6.   Mix thoroughly.

7.   Cover with the grated cheese & allow the cheese to melt.

8.   Serve on a plate of lettuce, rice/taco/burrito whether the cheese is melted!

21   Thai Red Curry Shrimp & Veggies

Servings: 4 | **Time:** 30 mins | **Difficulty:** Easy

Nutrients per serving: Calories: 368 kcal | Fat: 31g | Carbohydrates: 3g | Protein: 18g | Fiber: 1g

Ingredients

1.5 lb peeled raw wild-caught shrimp

1 large head riced cauliflower

2 Tbsp coconut oil (28g)

2 sliced shallots

4 big minced/pressed cloves garlic

2 sliced red bell peppers

2 peeled & thinly sliced stalks of lemongrass

6 sliced green onions

2 Tbsp freshly grated/finely minced ginger

1 can coconut milk full fat

1/2 cup organic chicken stock low sodium

2 Tbsp red curry paste

2 cups snap peas (250g)

8 Thai aubergines (135g)

2 small zested & juiced limes

1 small bunch of coriander

1 tsp fish sauce

Method

1.   Prepare the shrimp. Take the shrimp out of the fridge and pat it dry.

2.   Sauté rice with cauliflower. Heat 1 Tablespoon of coconut oil over med heat in the large pan. Sauté the cauliflower rice till tender but not fluffy (around 3 mins over med-high heat) (about 3 minutes over medium-high heat).

3.   Saute any veggies. In a wide pot, on med heat, heat the leftover 1 Tbsp of coconut oil. Put the garlic, shallot, red bell pepper, green onion & lemongrass (reserve some green onion for garnish). (reserve some green onion for garnish). Cook for six mins or till the veggies are tender, but they do not turn orange. Occasionally stir.

4.   Put curry paste & ginger. Cook for one min, sometimes stirring.

5.   Put the aubergine & liquids. Put coconut milk, chicken stock, fish sauce, & Thai aubergine. Carry & stir regularly to a boil, scraping the bottom & edges. For four mins, cook.

6.   Put snap peas & shrimp. Boil for around five min or till the shrimp is pink & opaque.

7.   Switch the heat off & put the lime juice & coriander to the mixture (reserve a few coriander for topping) (reserve some cilantro for garnish) (reserve some cilantro for garnish).

8. Sprinkle to taste

9. Garnish it. Serve with the additional green onions, cilantro, & lime zest on cauliflower rice & garnish.

22 Low Carb Beef Stroganoff Meatball

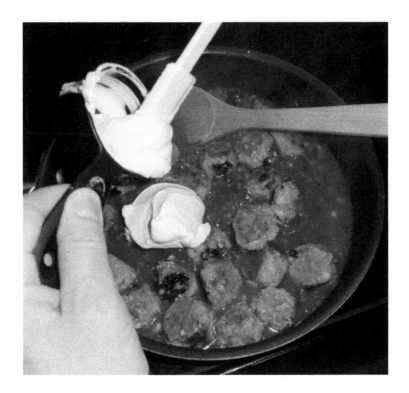

Servings: 4 | **Time**: 5 mins | **Difficulty**: Easy

Nutrients per serving: Calories: 452 kcal | Fat: 34g | Carbohydrates: 6g | Protein: 24g

Ingredients

For the meatball mix:

1 egg

1 lb ground beef

1 tsp kosher salt

1/4 cup almond flour

1/2 tsp garlic powder

1/2 tsp onion powder

1/4 tsp black pepper

1 tsp Worcestershire sauce

1 tsp dried parsley

2 Tbsp butter to fry

For the sauce:

2 cups sliced mushrooms

1 Tbsp butter

1 minced clove garlic

1 cup sliced onions

3/4 cup sour cream

1 1/2 cups beef broth

salt & pepper to taste

1/4 tsp xanthan gum

2 Tbsp chopped fresh parsley

Method

1.　　In a med bowl, mix the meatball components & combine well.

2.　　Form them into Twelve meatballs.

3.　　In a large, non-stick saute skillet, heat 2 Tablespoons of butter.

4.　　On med pressure, fry the meatballs in butter till browned on each side & cooked fully (2-3 minutes per side.)

5.　　Set aside & take the meatballs off the pan.

6.　　Put 1 tbsp of butter & two cups of mushroom slices in the skillet.

7.　　Cook till golden & fragrant mushrooms (4-5 minutes) (4-5 minutes.)

8.　　From the pan, remove the mushrooms.

9.　　Put the garlic & onions, then simmer for 3 to 4 mins, or till smooth & translucent.

10.　　From the pan, remove the onions.

11.　　To have all the yummy bits off, put the beef broth in the skillet & scrape a bottom.

12.　　Place the sour cream & xanthan gum & whisk till smooth.

13.　　Return to the skillet, put the mushrooms, meatballs, onions & garlic, then mix.

14.　　Boil for twenty mins at low.

15.　　Sprinkle with salt.

16.　　Right before eating, Top with the new parsley.

23   Low Carb Bacon Bok Choy

Servings: 2 | **Time:** 15 mins | **Difficulty:** Easy

Nutrients per serving: Calories: 154 kcal | Fat: 13g | Carbohydrates: 4g | Protein: 4g | Fiber: 1g

Ingredients

2 cups baby bok choy, chopped

2 slices pastured bacon

2 big cloves garlic

Method

1.   Start by frying the bacon in a pan. Take it from the pan & set it aside to cool when finished, retaining the pan's bacon grease.

2.   The garlic & the bok choy stems then cook for about 2-3 mins, stirring continuously to the pan.

3.   Put the leaves & stir till the leaves wilt.

4.   Enjoy & serve.

24   Korean Spicy Pork

Servings: 4 | **Time:** 40 mins | **Difficulty:** Easy

Nutrients per serving: Calories: 189 kcal | Fat: 9g | Carbohydrates: 9g | Protein: 15g | Fiber: 1g

Ingredients

For Marinating and Cooking:

1 lb Boneless Pork Shoulder

1 sliced Onion

1 tbsp Minced Ginger

1 tbsp Minced Garlic

1 tbsp Soy Sauce

1 tbsp rice wine

1 tbsp Sesame Oil

2 packets Splenda

2 tbsp gochujang

1/4-1 tsp Gochugaru

1/4 cup Water (62.5 ml)

For Finishing:

1 tbsp Sesame Seeds

1 Sliced Onion

1/4 cup Green Scallions, Chopped

Method

1.   Combine all the marinating & boiling supplies in the/ Instant Pot /Pressure Cooker's inner lining. If necessary, allow it to sit for at least an hour & up to 24 hrs.

2.   Cook for 20 mins at high pressure, then let it slowly relieve pressure for ten min. Release the residual pressure after ten minutes have gone.

3.   You can see the excellent meat & a yummy-looking sauce once you open the pot.

4.   Heat the pan.

5.   Put the cubes of pork & the finely diced onion in the hot skillet.

6.   Let it get warm, then place 1/4-1/2 cup of the sauce. This sauce can begin to sizzle & caramelize easily. Mix with the pork well.

7.   You attempt to evaporate this sauce, leave behind its delicious goodness on the meat.

8.   Drizzle with sesame seeds & green onions till the sauce has evaporated & the onions had softened & serve.

9.   To serve on the side, you should use the remainder of the sauce from the pressure cooker.

25 Prosciutto-Wrapped Cod with Lemon Caper Spinach

Servings: 2 | **Time**: 20 mins | **Difficulty:** Easy

Nutrients per serving: Calories: 660 kcal | Fat: 60g | Carbohydrates: 7g | Protein: 13g | Fiber: 7g

Ingredients

4 cups of baby spinach

2 Tbsps. of ghee, or grass-fed butter, or avocado oil

1 tsp. of lemon juice (fresh)

Salt & freshly ground black pepper

1 lemons' zest

12 to 14 oz. of cod fillets

1 minced clove of garlic

1.5 oz. of prosciutto de Parma

2 Tbsps. of capers

Method

1.   With paper towels, dry the fish fillets completely, and thaw them (if frozen) for half an hour until they reach room temperature.

2.   After they have come to room temperature, dry them again if necessary. Sprinkle the fillets with salt and freshly ground black pepper. Please keep in mind; prosciutto also has salt in it.

3.   Gently Wrap the prosciutto around seasoned fish fillets, so they would not tear up.

4.   Lay prosciutto's strips into a sheet on a flat surface, if they are in strips, and then wrap the fish fillets.

5.   In a cast-iron skillet, on medium flame, melt ghee or butter or the oil you are using.

6.   Place prosciutto-wrapped fish fillets in skillet and let them cook, until fish flakes with a fork easily, for five minutes on each side

7.   It will take you about ten minutes to cook. Although this cooking time is for fillet (one-inch thickness), it may vary depending upon fish fillets' thickness and size.

8.   Cook until the meat thermometer shows 140 F or 160 C.

9.   Take the fillets out and let them cool on a wire rack. Keeping them on the rack will not let the bottom get soggy.

10.   Add minced garlic to the used pan, and sauté for half a minute.

11.   Add capers, lemon juice, and spinach.

12.   Keep mixing and cook for two minutes, or until the spinach wilts.

13.   Take spinach mix out on serving plates, place fish on top, and drizzle lemon juice and zest.

14.   Serve right away and enjoy.

26   Creamy Shrimp & Bacon skillet

Servings: 4 | **Time:** 10 mins | **Difficulty**: Easy

Nutrients per serving: Calories: 340 kcal | Fat: 29g | Carbohydrates: 3.5g | Protein: 17g | Fiber: 1g

Ingredients

4 oz. of smoked salmon

Half cup of coconut cream

1 cup of mushrooms, sliced

4 oz. of shelled raw shrimp

Freshly ground black pepper, to taste

1 pinch of Sea Salt

4 slices of uncured bacon (organic)

Method

1.   Slice the bacon into one-inch pieces

2.   In a cast-iron skillet, add bacon pieces to the skillet, cook on medium heat for almost five minutes.

3.   Do not make the bacon crispy; slightly cook it, add mushrooms slices sauté for five more minutes.

4.   Cut the smoked salmon in strips, and add in the mushrooms, cook for 2-4 minutes

5.   Add raw shrimps and cook for almost two minutes on high heat.

6.   Add in the salt and cream, turn the heat low, and cook for 60 seconds, or until the sauce becomes thick enough for your liking.

7.   Serve right away with zucchini noodles if you like.

27 One-Pot Chicken Cacciatore

Servings: 6 | **Time:** 1 hour | **Difficulty**: Medium

Nutrients per serving: Calories: 451 kcal | Fat: 23g | Carbohydrates: 24g | Protein: 29g | Fiber: 4g

Ingredients

28 oz. of crushed tomatoes

1 cup of White wine

2 Chicken breasts skin on, bone-in,

1 bell pepper (red), cut into slices

4 thighs of Chicken, or skin on drumsticks & thighs both, bone-in Half cup of all-purpose Flour

1 and a half tsp. of Salt, add more to taste

1 bell pepper (green), cut into slices

2 tbsps. of Olive oil

1 sliced Onion, large-sized

1 tsp. of freshly ground black pepper

3/4 cup of Chicken Broth

2 cups of Mushrooms, cut into slices

2 minced cloves of garlic

Method

1.   Season the chicken with salt and freshly ground black pepper.

2.   Coat the seasoned chicken in all-purpose chicken.

3.   In a Dutch oven, add olive oil, brown the chicken in batches on a medium flame for three minutes for each side.

4.   Take the chicken out and place it on a plate, set it aside.

5.   In the pot, add garlic, peppers, mushrooms, half tsp. of salt and onions, cook for 2 to 3 minutes.

6.   Add the white wine and let it simmer, cook until it is reduced by half.

7.   Add broth, one tsp. of salt, and tomatoes to the pot.

8.   Add the chicken in sauce in the pot.

9.   With the lid on, let it simmer.

10.   Cook for almost half an hour until the chicken is tender and cooked through.

11.   Serve with bread or over rice or pasta to your liking.

28 Texas Chicken Nachos

Servings: 4 | **Time:** 20 mins | **Difficulty:** Easy

Nutrients per serving: Calories: 660 kcal | Fat: 60g | Carbohydrates: 7g | Protein: 13g | Fiber: 7g

Ingredients

1 and a half tsp. of smoked paprika

1 and a half cups of cheddar cheese

3 tbsp. of green onion

1 and a half lbs. of chicken tenders

3/4 tsp. of chili powder

1 tbsp. of olive oil

1 and a half tsp. of kosher salt

6 bacon slices, cooked & crumbled

Half tsp. of cayenne pepper

1 jalapeno

3/4 tsp. of cumin

Method

1.   Let the oven preheat to 350 F.

2.   In a bowl, mix paprika, cumin, salt, cayenne pepper, and chili powder.

3.   Coat the chicken pieces well in the spice rub. Add olive oil on spice coated chicken and distribute the oil well over chicken.

4.   Place the seasoned chicken pieces on a baking sheet and do not overcrowd the baking sheet leaving at least half an inch of space between chicken pieces.

5.   Bake for 3 to 4 minutes at 350 F, flip the chicken pieces once and bake for another 3 to 4 minutes.

6.   Add jalapeno and cheese to the chicken. Place back in the oven and bake at 425 F until cheese melts for almost 3 to 4 minutes.

7.   Take out from the oven and garnish with bacon and green onion on top.

8.   Serve right away, or serve with blue cheese dressing or ranch dressing.

29 Keto Cheesy Spinach Stuffed Chicken Breast

Servings: 4 | **Time:** 55 mins | **Difficulty:** Medium

Nutrients per serving: Calories: 491 kcal | Fat: 33g | Carbohydrates: 3.5g | Protein: 43g

Ingredients

Half tsp. of minced garlic

2 cups of chopped spinach

4 skinless chicken cutlets or breasts, boneless

1/3 cup of parmesan cheese (grated)

6 oz. of softened cream cheese

1/4 tsp. of kosher salt

Half cup of mozzarella cheese (grated)

1/8 tsp. of ground nutmeg

1/4 tsp. of freshly ground black pepper

For the breading:

1/8 tsp. of garlic powder

1/3 cup of parmesan cheese (grated)

1/8 tsp. of onion powder

Half tsp. of dried parsley

1/3 cup of superfine almond flour

2 tbsp. of olive oil

2 whole eggs

Half tsp. of kosher salt

Method

1.   In a bowl, mix garlic, cream cheese, freshly ground black pepper, nutmeg, salt, parmesan, spinach, and mozzarella. Mix well and set it aside.

2.   Clean the chicken if any visible membrane or fat is present.

3.   (If chicken breasts are large, then slice them in half lengthwise and flatten them, so use 2 of chicken breasts cut into four pieces).

4.   On a clean surface, place one layer of plastic wrap and wrap one piece of chicken in plastic wrap.

5.   Flatten the chicken by pounding with a mallet, from one side to the center. Do not flatten it too much so that it may become very thin.

6.   Repeat the process on all chicken pieces.

7.   Place ¼ of spinach mixture in the center of chicken pieces and roll them tightly.

8.   Seal the edges with your clean hands. So, the filling will not get out.

9.   On a baking sheet, place all pieces of chicken seam side down.

10.   Keep in the fridge for 15 minutes.

11.   In a bowl, whisk the eggs.

12.   In another bowl, mix all the ingredients of breading and mix well (do not add olive oil).

13.   In a cast-iron skillet, heat the olive oil.

14.   Let the oven preheat to 375 F.

15.   Coat the chicken in the whisked egg, then in breading, then fry in oil on all sides until light brown.

16.   Place the chicken on a baking pan.

17.   Bake for 18 to 22 minutes, at 375 F, or until internal temperature shows 165 F.

18.   Serve with alfredo sauce or rice.

30 Low Carb Muffuletta Chicken

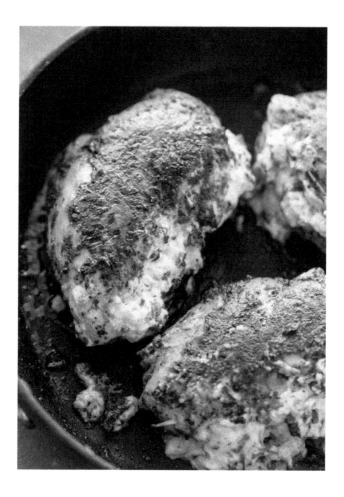

Servings: 4 | **Time:** 25 mins | **Difficulty:** Easy

Nutrients per serving: Calories: 846 kcal | Fat: 64g | Carbohydrates: 6g | Protein: 57g | Fiber: 1g

Ingredients

Muffuletta Chicken

4 oz. of mortadella, cut into slices

1 and a half lb. of chicken breasts

4 oz. of salami, cut into thin slices

4 oz. of capocollo, cut into thin slices

2 cups of Olive Salad

4 oz. of provolone cheese, cut into slices

¼ cup of butter (half of the stick)

4 oz. of mozzarella cheese, cut into slices

For Chicken:

1 cup of green olives

Half tsp of freshly ground black pepper

1 and a half cups of Giardiniera vegetables (pickled)

1 tsp. of dried oregano

⅓ cup of red wine vinegar

¼ cup of olive oil

4 large garlic cloves

Half cup of pepperoncini

1 cup of Kalamata olives

¼ cup of red peppers (roasted)

Half cup of capers

1 tsp. of dried basil

Method

1.   Sear the chicken breast: add butter in a skillet, over medium flame, and cook chicken for 8 minutes on every side until light brown.

2.   Let the oven preheat to 350 F.

3.   In a rimmed cookie sheet, add chicken and layer the chicken with capocollo, provolone, mozzarella, salami, and mortadella.

4.   Bake for ten minutes on the middle rack.

5.   Take chicken out of the oven, add the olive salad on top, and serve right away.

For Olive Salad:

1.   Add the garlic, Kalamata olives, olive oil, pickled vegetables, pepperoncini, roasted red peppers, red wine vinegar, and green olives in a food processor.

2.   Pulse until roughly chopped.

3.   Add in freshly ground black pepper, oregano, and basil. Pulse until combined.

4.   Add in the capers. Keep in the fridge for at least 60 minutes before serving with chicken

31 Pistachio Crusted Salmon

Servings: 4 | **Time:** 20 mins | **Difficulty:** Easy

Nutrients per serving: Calories: 298 kcal | Fat: 18g | Carbohydrates: 6g | Protein: 27g | Fiber: 2g

Ingredients

Salt and freshly ground black pepper, to taste

3 tbsp. of Dijon mustard

3/4 cup of Pistachios, finely diced

16 oz. of Salmon

Method

1.   Let the oven preheat to 400F.

2.   Season the salmon with salt and freshly ground black pepper.

3.   Spread mustard on every filet, and press in finely cut pistachios.

4.   Put on an oiled baking pan and bake at 400 F for 10 to 15 minutes, until fish flakes easily and tender.

5.   Serve right away and enjoy.

32   Grouper Caprese

Servings: 4 | **Time:** 25 mins | **Difficulty**: Easy

Nutrients per serving: Calories: 442 kcal | Fat: 18g | Carbohydrates: 3g | Protein: 63g

Ingredients

2 Roma Tomatoes, cut into thin slices

8 oz. of grated Mozzarella

Salt and freshly ground Black Pepper

4 Grouper fillets

2 tbsp. of Pesto

Method

1.   Let the oven preheat to 350 F.

2.   Season the Grouper with salt and freshly ground black pepper.

3.   Fry in a skillet for two minutes on every side.

4.   Put on a baking sheet.

5.   Rub each side with pesto, add 3 to 4 thin slices of tomatoes, top with grated cheese.

6.   Bake for eight minutes in the oven. Serve right away.

33 Roasted Shrimp with Lemon & Herb Spaghetti Squash

Servings: 4 | **Time:** 70 mins | **Difficulty:** Difficult

Nutrients per serving: Calories: 235 kcal | Fat: 10.4g | Carbohydrates: 25.7g | Protein: 9.7g | Fiber: 4.3g

Ingredients

12 oz. of peeled large shrimp, deveined

2 tbsp. of grass-fed butter

¼ cup of plain Greek yogurt

Juice of one lemon

Salt & freshly ground black pepper, to taste

Half cup of dry white wine

1 tbsp. of olive oil

¼ tsp. of red pepper flakes

3 minced cloves of garlic

1 tsp. of lemon zest

2 spaghetti squash, small sized

2 tbsp. of chopped parsley, fresh

1 tsp. of Dijon mustard

Method

1.   Let the oven preheat to 350 F, cut the squash in half lengthwise, take all the seeds out.

2.   Put the middle side squash down on an oiled baking sheet.

3.   Bake for 45 minutes at 350 F, till squash is tender.

4.   In a skillet, add butter and oil on medium flame. Season the shrimp with freshly ground black pepper and salt and sauté in butter oil mixture for almost two minutes.

5.   Add garlic and sauté for another two minutes until the shrimp is completely cooked, but do not overcook the shrimp. Turn off the heat and set it aside.

6.   Add Dijon mustard, lemon juice, red pepper flakes, white wine, and lemon zest. Let it boil. Turn the heat low and let it simmer till the squash has completely baked. Turn off the heat.

7.   Take the squash out of the oven. With a fork, scrape out the spaghetti flesh.

8.   Add spaghetti squash in a strainer and let the excess water drip, carefully press with a paper towel.

9.   Add yogurt in sauce, till smooth and creamy. Add in chopped fresh parsley.

10.   Coat the spaghetti squash in shrimp and sauce and serve.

34 Skillet Salmon with Avocado & Basil

Servings: 4 | **Time:** 15 mins | **Difficulty:** Easy

Nutrients per serving: Calories: 232 kcal | Fat: 9g | Carbohydrates: 7g | Protein: 32g | Fiber: 3g

Ingredients

1 and a half pounds of skinless salmon filet, boneless

2 tsp. of coconut oil

1 tbsp. of lime juice

Half tsp. of crushed red pepper

1 tsp. of Italian seasoning

¼ tsp. of freshly ground black pepper

1 and a half tsp. of kosher salt

One whole avocado

For garnish, sliced scallions

¼ cup of chopped basil

Method

1.   In a cast-iron skillet, add oil on medium flame.

2. Season the salmon with crushed red pepper, ¾ tsp. of salt, freshly ground black pepper, Italian seasonings.

3. Place the seasoned salmon filet in oil.

4. Let it cook, do not flip until crispy and browned along the edge, cook for 4-6 minutes. Cooking time depends on thickness.

5. Flip the fish over and turn off the heat.

6. Let it cook on the other side in the heated skillet, for about four minutes or until cooked to your liking.

7. Peel and pit the avocado and mix with the rest of the salt, lime juice, and basil.

8. Serve salmon with avocado mash.

9. Top with sliced scallions and serve.

35 Cedar Plank Grilled Fish

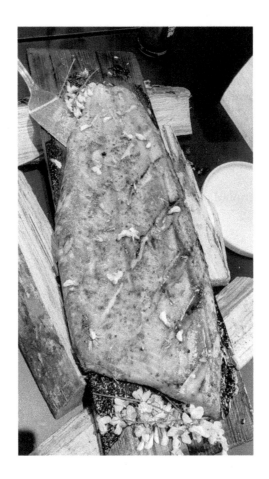

Servings: 2 | **Time:** 20 mins | **Difficulty**: Easy

Nutrients per serving: Calories: 147 kcal | Fat: 5g | Carbohydrates: 2g | Protein: 23g

Ingredients

1 pinch of paprika

1 Cedar plank

1 Lemon, thinly sliced

1 pinch of garlic powder

3 parsley sprigs

1 to 2 pounds of cleaned Fish

1 pinch of freshly ground black pepper

1 tbsp. of olive oil

1 pinch of salt

Method

1.   Let the grill preheat to high.

2.   Pre-soak the plank and coat with olive oil.

3.   Place the fish on the plank.

4.   Season the inside of the fish with paprika, salt, garlic powder, and freshly ground black pepper.

5.   Stuff the fish with parsley and thin slices of lemon.

6.   Grill for 10 to 14 minutes on the covered grill.

7.   Serve right away.

36 Balsamic Glazed Rosemary Steak Skewers

Servings: 6 | **Time:** 36 mins | **Difficulty**: Easy

Nutrients per serving: Calories: 660 kcal | Fat: 60g | Carbohydrates: 7g | Protein: 13g | Fiber: 7g

Ingredients

Fresh Rosemary, thick stalks

1-pound of Grape or cherry tomatoes

Marinade

2 and a half pounds of Sirloin steak, slice into 1 and a half-inch cubes

1 tsp. of Salt

¼ cup of Balsamic glaze

1 tsp. of Dijon mustard

¾ cup of Vegetable oil

Method

1.   In a bowl, add all ingredients of the marinade and add in a zip-lock bag.

2.   Add beef to the bag and coat well. Keep in the fridge for 60 minutes or more.

3.   Take leaves of rosemary stalks and leave some on the top.

4.   Thread the meat on rosemary skewers with tomatoes and beef.

5.   Repeat the process until the meat is gone.

6.   Grill the meat for three minutes on every side until tender.

37   Balsamic Steak Roll-Ups

Servings: 4 | **Time:** 1 hour 10 mins | **Difficulty:** Easy

Nutrients per serving: Calories: 327 kcal | Fat: 12g | Carbohydrates: 12g | Protein: 39g | Fiber: 3g

Ingredients

Half cup of Balsamic Vinegar (Aged)

freshly ground black pepper, to taste

1 and a half pounds of Sirloin or Flank Steak

2 to 3 Carrots

Salt, to taste

Olive Oil, as needed

1 pound of Asparagus

Method

1.   Slice the steak into three-inch of strips.

2.   Place every piece in plastic wrap and pound with a mallet to 1/4 inch of thickness.

3.   Put the steak in a dish and pour balsamic vinegar on top, cover with plastic wrap, let it rest for 1 to 2 hours.

4.   Season the steak with freshly ground black pepper and salt.

5.   Wrap the trimmed asparagus bunch in a moist paper towel and microwave for two minutes.

6.   Slice carrots into thin pieces.

7.   Wrap the vegetables in meat and make a roll, secure with a toothpick.

8.   Make all meat rolls with vegetables.

9.   In a pan, add olive oil and add steak rolls and cook for 1 to 2 minutes on each side.

10.   Let it rest for five minutes before serving.

38   Greek Chicken Roll-Ups

Servings: 4 | **Time**: 30 mins | **Difficulty**: Easy

Nutrients per serving: Calories: 660 kcal | Fat: 60g | Carbohydrates: 7g | Protein: 13g | Fiber: 7g

Ingredients

2 Chicken Breasts, cut in halves

Salt, to taste

4 oz. of softened Cream Cheese

Half cup of Black Ripe Olives, chopped

4 oz. of Feta Cheese

Method

1.   Let the oven preheat to 400 F.

2.   Pound the chicken breast in plastic wrap with a mallet until they all are the same thickness.

3.   In a bowl, mix ripe olives, cream cheese, and feta cheese.

4.   Add 2 to 3 tbsp. of olive mix into every chicken breast piece and roll it up.

5.   Put all rolls in an oiled baking pan—Bake for 20 to 30 minutes.

6.   Serve right away and enjoy.

39 Almond Parmesan Baked Salmon

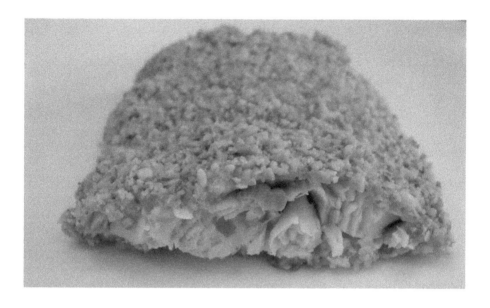

Servings: 1 | **Time:** 20 mins | **Difficulty**: Easy

Nutrients per serving: Calories: 412.8 kcal | Fat: 29.19g | Carbohydrates: 3.5g | Protein: 34.34g | Fiber: 1.48g

Ingredients

1 bunch of cilantro

3/4 cup of almond flour

1/3 cup of melted butter

Salt & freshly ground black pepper, to taste

3/4 cup of Parmesan cheese (grated)

1 salmon fillet

Method

1.   Let the oven preheat to 400 F.

2.   Trim and clean the cilantro, cut the stems. Chop the cilantro leaves.

3.   In a bowl, add almond flour, chopped cilantro, melted butter, and parmesan. Mix with a fork.

4.   Place a baking paper on a baking sheet, place fish skin side down, and season with freshly ground black pepper and salt.

5.   Coat the fish with parmesan mix and press with your hands on the fish.

6.   Bake at 400 F for 15 minutes.

7.   Serve and enjoy.

40   Keto Creamy Cajun Chicken

Servings: 6 | **Time:** 35 mins | **Difficulty**: Easy

Nutrients per serving: Calories: 547 kcal | Fat: 39g | Carbohydrates: 5g | Protein: 42g | Fiber: 1g

Ingredients

1 cup of grated parmesan

2 tbsp. of butter

2 tbsp. of avocado oil

Blackened Seasoning

2 lbs. of chicken breasts, cut into cutlets

1 onion, cut into slices

1 and a half cup of heavy cream

3 green onions, cut into slices

1 bell pepper, cut into slices

1 and a half cup of chicken broth

2 minced cloves of garlic

Method

1.   Season the chicken with blackened seasoning generously and set it aside.

2.   In a skillet, add avocado oil and butter on medium flame.

3.   Sear the chicken in batches for 3 to 4 minutes on each side until the chicken's internal temperature reaches 165 F.

4.   Use a smoke vent if smoke is too much.

5.   Cut the chicken into slices.

6.   Add pepper and onion to the pan, cook for 2 to 3 minutes.

7.   Add garlic and cook for 60 seconds more.

8.   Add chicken stock to the pan and let it boil. Turn the heat low, and let it simmer for 8 to ten minutes, reduce it by half.

9.   Add cream and let it simmer until it also reduces by half and becomes thick.

10.   Turn the heat low, add in the cheese. Mix until cheese melts.

11.   Add sliced chicken back into the sauce with its juices.

12.   Serve with cheese and green onion on top.

41   Bacon Wrapped Chicken Diablos

Servings: 6 | **Time:** 40 mins | **Difficulty:** Easy

Nutrients per serving: Calories: 660 kcal | Fat: 60g | Carbohydrates: 7g | Protein: 13g | Fiber: 7g

Ingredients

Six slices of smoked bacon

3 jalapenos, cut into halves, seeds removed

Half purple or sweet onion, slice into 4 to 5 wedges

6 oz. of Pepper Jack Cheese, cut into 6 slices

2 to 3 chicken breast, horizontally cut into thin slices Your preferred seasoning rub, as needed

Method

1.   Season the chicken generously with seasoning. Season the onion and peppers too.

2.   Place one chicken piece on a clean surface, add cheese, onion pieces on chicken with jalapeno cut side down over cheese.

3.   Roll the chicken tightly with cheese, onion, and pepper inside. With bacon, wrap around the chicken roll and close with a toothpick.

4.   Keep repeating for all slices of chicken breast.

5.   Now, either keep these in the fridge in a closed container or cook them right away.

6.   Let the grill heat up for 15 to 20 minutes to 350 to 400 F. Grill the chicken until it is completely cooked and cheese melts.

7.   You can bake the chicken at 400 F for 15 to 20 minutes.

8.   Cooking time depends upon the thickness of chicken pieces.

42 Roasted Red Pepper & Caramelized Onion Frittata

Servings: 8-10 | **Time:** 1 hr | **Difficulty:** Medium

Nutrients per serving: Calories: 660 kcal | Fat: 60g | Carbohydrates: 7g | Protein: 13g | Fiber: 7g

Ingredients

1 and a half cup of shredded Fontina cheese

1 tbsp. of butter

Half cup of roasted bell pepper (2 peppers)

2 tsp. of salt

1 tsp. of freshly ground black pepper

12 whole eggs

Half cup of sour cream

2 sweet onions, large-size, cut into halves and ¼" strips

Method

1.   Let the oven preheat to 350 F.

2.   In a cast-iron skillet, melt the butter on medium flame, and saute onions for 40 minutes or until caramelized and soft.

3.   Meanwhile, whisk the eggs with sour cream, salt, freshly ground black pepper, cheese. Mix well, but do not over whisk the eggs.

4.   Spread the caramelized onions in the pan in one layer. Add roasted red pepper on caramelized onions.

5.   Pour the whisked eggs over onion and peppers. Cook for 3 to 5 minutes on low flame just as eggs start to set.

6.   Place the pan in the oven and bake for 15 to 17 minutes. Eggs should have a custard-like consistency.

7.   Make sure to use an oven-proof skillet, and I used a 12" skillet.

8.   Serve and enjoy.

43 Poached Cod in Tomato Sauce

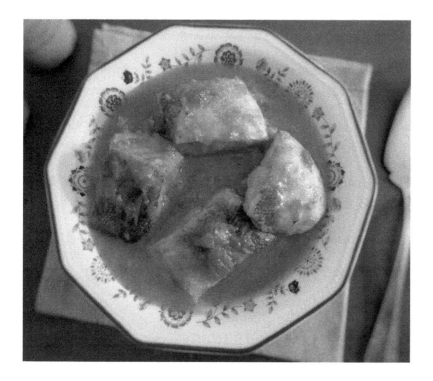

Servings: 4 | **Time:** 25 mins | **Difficulty:** Easy

Nutrients per serving: Calories: 169 kcal | Fat: 1g | Carbohydrates: 7g | Protein: 34g | Fiber: 2g

Ingredients

Kosher or sea salt, to taste

2 cups of marinara sauce

4 skinless & boneless cod fillets (6-oz.)

¼ cup of fresh herbs (chopped) such as basil, chives, cilantro, or Italian parsley

Freshly ground black pepper, to taste

Method

1.   Thaw the cod the whole night in the fridge if the fish is frozen. Or keep in cool water for 10 to 15 minutes.

2.   With paper towels, dry the fish and season with salt.

3.   In a ten-inch skillet, add 2 cups of marinara sauce. Fish should fit in one single layer in the skillet.

4.   Keep the skillet on medium flame and boil the sauce. As the sauce is boiling, add fish into the sauce.

5.   Turn the heat low, and let it simmer.

6.   Cover the skillet and let it cook for 5-8 minutes or until fish flakes easily.

7.   The internal temperature of fish should be 130 to 140 F with a meat thermometer.

8.   Sprinkle fresh herbs and freshly ground black pepper on fish.

9.   Serve right away with rice or sautéed vegetables.

44 Instant Pot Zucchini Bolognese

Servings: 4 | **Time:** 1 hr | **Difficulty:** Difficult

Nutrients per serving: Calories: 498 kcal | Fat: 43g | Carbohydrates: 9g | Protein: 19g | Fiber: 2g

Ingredients

3 minced cloves of garlic

1 yellow, large-sized onion, diced

2 tbsp. of avocado oil or olive oil

1 and a half pounds of zucchini chopped into half" pieces

1 pound of Italian sausage (bulk)

Juice from half lemon

Magic Mushroom Powder, 1 tsp.

Method

1.   Turn on the function of sauteing in the instant pot, then add in the olive oil.

2.   Add in the chopped onion and cook for 2-3 minutes, keep stirring, until onion softens.

3.   Add sausage and break it up with a spoon. Cook until it is cooked through.

4.   Add in garlic, zucchini, magic mushroom powder. Mix it well.

5.   Do not add any liquid; zucchini will have some liquid of its own.

6.   Lock the instant pot, and cook for 35 minutes under high pressure.

7.   Let the pressure release on its own, or manually vent.

8.   Vegetables should be soft; mash with a spoon to make the sauce chunky.

9.   Taste and adjust the seasoning of the sauce with salt, black pepper, or mushroom powder.

10.   Add in the lemon juice. Season it again if required.

11.   Make the noodles from zucchini in a spiralizer. Add the spiralized noodles to the sauce and coat them well.

12.   Sprinkle with herbs and serve.

13.   You can freeze the sauce also, for later use.

45 Lemon Garlic Chicken Parchment Packets

Servings: 4 | **Time:** 30 mins | **Difficulty**: Medium

Nutrients per serving: Calories: 425 kcal | Fat: 27g | Carbohydrates: 11g | Protein: 36g | Fiber: 3g

Ingredients

2 minced garlic cloves

⅓ cup of olive oil

Freshly cracked black pepper, to taste

¼ cup of lemon juice (freshly squeezed)

1 shallot large-size cut into thin slices

Kosher salt, to taste

4 skinless chicken boneless breasts or thighs (almost 6 oz. each)

1 and a half tsp. of dried oregano

8 tomatoes (cherry) slice in half

4 summer squash medium-sized, cut into thin coin

8 green olives, pitted, sliced in half

Method

1.   Let the oven preheat to 450 F.

2.   In a bowl, mix kosher salt, olive oil, ¼ tsp. freshly ground black pepper, lemon juice, oregano, and minced garlic.

3.   Add the meat and coat well, and let it rest for ten minutes or 2 hours. Do not marinate for more than that.

4.   Take four sheets of parchment paper and double in half. Make one side of the heart on it. Cut it so one will get full hearts.

5.   Lay these hearts on a flat surface. Add ¼ of Zucchini or summer squash on each side of the heart. Add onion rings to it and season with freshly ground black pepper and salt.

6.   Put one chicken piece over the vegetables, and pour 2 tbsp. of the marinade on the chicken.

7.   Add ¼ of cherry tomatoes and olives over them. Do the same for the rest of the packets.

8.   Place the other half of the heart over the chicken and fold the edges tightly.

9.   On a baking sheet, place the packets in one layer.

10.   Bake for 15 to 20 minutes, until the internal temperature of the chicken shows 165 F.

11.   Cut the packet to release the steam and serve right away and enjoy.

46   Rack of Lamb

Servings: 4 | **Time:** 1 day 55 mins | **Difficulty:** Difficult

Nutrients per serving: Calories: 417 kcal | Fat: 32g | Carbohydrates: 3g | Protein: 30g | Fiber: 1g

Ingredients

4 minced cloves of garlic

2 lamb racks French cut almost 1 and a half pounds of each rack

⅓ cup of olive oil (extra virgin)

Half tsp. of freshly cracked black pepper

3 tbsp. of lemon juice

2 tsp. of kosher salt

1 tbsp. of oregano (dried)

Method

1.   Clean the extra fat from the rack of lamb, only leave a thin layer.

2.   Coat the rack of lamb in salt and keep it in the fridge overnight or for 3 days.

3.   In a bowl, mix garlic, freshly cracked black pepper, olive oil, lemon juice, and oregano.

4.   Coat the rack of lamb in marinade mix and keep in the fridge for 1 to 12 hours.

5.   Let the oven preheat to 275 F, put the marinated rack of lamb on a baking sheet, and place in the middle rack in the oven.

6.   Bake for 30 to 45 minutes, for medium-rare, until internal temperature shows 125°F.

7.   Take the meat out and turn the broiler on to the highest temperature.

8.   Broil the rack of lamb for five minutes, so the outside is browned well.

9.   Slice and serve the meat after 10 minutes of resting the meat.

47 Crab & Avocado Temaki

Servings: 4 | **Time:** 20 mins | **Difficulty**: Easy

Nutrients per serving: Calories: 256 kcal | Fat: 15g | Carbohydrates: 7g | Protein: 23g | Fiber: 4g

Ingredients

1 pound of lump crab meat (cooked)

2 small size cucumbers slice into thin pieces

Freshly cracked black pepper, to taste

8 nori sheets (toasted)

1 avocado large-sized, peeled & pitted, cut into thin slices

2 tbsp. of mayonnaise (paleo)

Half tsp. of red pepper flakes (it is optional)

2 scallions cut into thin slices

One and a half tbsp. of sesame seeds (toasted)

1 tbsp. of lime juice

Diamond Crystal Kosher salt, to taste

1 cup of microgreens

Method

1.   If you are busy and want to prepare this dish quickly, then skip this next step, but if you have time, make sure to follow it because even toasted nori sheets taste amazing when heated.

2.   Heat every sheet of nori on the gas burner on medium to low flame, gradually fan it back and forth until they become bright green.

3.   If one does not have a gas burner, make sure to use the oven. Switch on the broiler

and place the rack almost six inches away from the heating source. Put 2 sheets of nori on the rimmed baking sheet and place them in the oven for about ten seconds or till they turn green and smell fragrant.

4.   Slice every toasted sheet of nori in two pieces so that one will have 16 pieces of nori sheets that are toasted.

5.   In a mixing bowl, add the mayonnaise, crab meat, lime juice, red pepper flakes, and scallions. Taste and adjust seasoning with salt and freshly ground black pepper to your liking. Mix well and set it aside.

6.   To make nori rolls, place a piece of nori, shiny side down and place 2 tbsp. of crab mix on nori piece and, filling needs to be diagonal, from the top side of left to the center of the bottom of the sheet.

7.   Add the slice of avocado on top of crab meat, sprouts, and cucumber. Roll the sheet around the vegetables and crab meat in a shape to make a cone.

8.   Add sesame seeds on top; toast them if they are not toasted.

9.   Serve right away so the nori will not get soft, and you will get crispy bites of nori vegetable crab meat rolls.

48 Pork Stew Instant Pot

Servings: 6 | **Time:** 1 hr | **Difficulty**: Difficult

Nutrients per serving: Calories: 335 kcal | Fat: 14g | Carbohydrates: 15g | Protein: 35g | Fiber: 6g

Ingredients

3 and a half pounds of pork shoulder, sliced into 1 and a half-inch of cubes

1 onion large-sized, cut into thin slices

6 cloves of garlic peeled & smashed

1 tbsp. of olive oil (extra virgin) or ghee or avocado oil

1 tbsp. of balsamic vinegar (aged)

1 tbsp. of Mushroom Magic Powder or Crystal ¼ cup of Italian parsley, finely chopped, it is optional

3 carrots, medium size, cut into two-inch of chunks

1 cup of marinara sauce

1 cabbage, small size, cut into eight wedges

Diamond Crystal kosher salt, to taste

Freshly ground black pepper, to taste

1 tsp. of fish sauce (Red Boat)

Method

1.   In the instant pot, Turn on the function of sautéing. As the inserted metal gets hot, add in the oil of your choice.

2.   Add in onions, and saute till tender or fragrant.

3.   Add in the smashed garlic and keep stirring until fragrant, for almost 30 seconds. Make sure not to burn it.

4.   Add in the pieces of pork, and add the fish sauce and Mushroom magic powder.

5.   Make sure to mix well to season the meat.

6.   Add in marinara sauce over the top of the cubed pork pieces, do not mix it. Maybe a few of the recent Instant Pots will tell you a "Burn" message (error) if the marina sauce starts to scald.

7.   Now switch off the function of sautéing. Cook for 30 to 35 minutes with the lid locked and on high pressure.

8.   As the pork gets done cooking. Let the pressure release manually or let it release naturally; it is your choice.

9.   Add cabbage and the carrots to the instant pot and cook for three minutes on high pressure

10.   Again release the pressure naturally or manually and add in the aged balsamic vinegar.

11.   Taste and adjust the seasoning of the stew and adjust with freshly ground

black pepper and salt if required.

12.   Garnish the stew with Italian parsley freshly chopped. Serve and enjoy.

49   Sonoran Hot Dogs

Servings: 4 | **Time**: 30 mins | **Difficulty**: Easy

Nutrients per serving: Calories: 263 kcal | Fat: 19g | Carbohydrates: 13g | Protein: 12g | Fiber: 5g

Ingredients

4 sugar-free hot dogs if you are on a Whole30

8 lettuce butter leaves

1 bell pepper (red) or other colors, cut into thin slices

1 Hass avocado large size, peeled & cut into thin slices

1 onion, large size, cut into thin slices

4 slices of bacon sugar-free if you are on a Whole30

Crystal Diamond kosher salt

Half cup of pico de gallo or salsa of your choice

Method

1.   Wrap every hot dog in one strip of sugar-free bacon in one later, tuck the bacon strips' ends so it would not get open every time.

2.   Take a 12-inch cast-iron skillet and place it on medium flame. As it gets hot, put hot dogs wrapped in bacon strips in the center of the skillet.

3.   Pan-fry the bacon-wrapped hot dogs until the bacon becomes browned. Flip to the other side and brown on the other side as well.

4.   Add in the bell peppers and onions all over the hot dogs and in any space available.

5.   Season with salt, vegetables, and hot dogs.

6.   Keep browning the bacon-wrapped hot dogs, onions, and bell peppers, to make sure they cook evenly.

7.   It will be ready when bacon is browned and slightly crispy, onion and bell peppers are caramelized and tender.

8.   Serve these bacon-wrapped hot dogs, onion, and bell pepper in lettuce butter leaves.

9.   Garnish with your choice of salsa or pico de gallo and thinly cut avocado slices.

10.   Serve and enjoy.

50   Vegetable Soup in Instant Pot

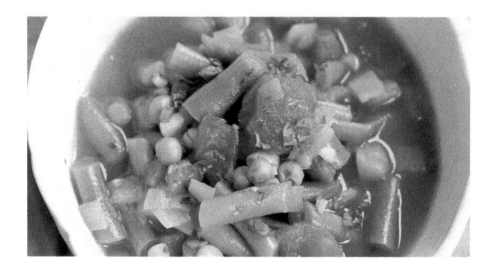

Servings: 4 | **Time**: 15 mins | **Difficulty**: Easy

Nutrients per serving: Calories: 205 kcal | Fat: 1g | Carbohydrates: 14g | Protein: 39g | Fiber: 4g

Ingredients

1 russet potato, medium-sized, cut into one inch of cubes

6 cups of Bone Broth or chicken broth (Instant Pot)

1 shallot, large-sized, cut into thin slices

2 carrots, medium-sized, peeled & cut into ¼ inch of coins

3 shiitake mushrooms (dried)

1 tsp. of fish sauce (Red Boat)

2 scallions cut into thin slices

1 pound of baby bok choy trim the ends, & cut in half or in quartered, if too large

2 minced cloves of garlic

Crystal Diamond kosher salt

Method

1.   In the instant pot, add in the bone broth when the metal insert turns hot.

2.   Add in the shallots, carrots, and potatoes. Do not splash yourself. Add in fish sauce (red boat), shiitake mushrooms, and garlic. Add in the quartered bok choy.

3.   Cook for 2 minutes, with the lid locked of instant pot on high pressure.

4.   As the soup gets done cooking, release the pressure naturally or manually, your choice.

5.   Taste and adjust seasoning with fish sauce and salt as needed.

6.   Take the soup out in the bowl, garnish with scallions.

7.   Serve and enjoy this delicious soup.

Lightning Source UK Ltd.
Milton Keynes UK
UKHW020703070922
408471UK00010B/960